RECLAIMING MY TIME

A Black Woman's Guide to Self-Care

Dr. Tiffany M Jenkins

Awakening Change Publishing
A Subsidiary of
Awakening Change Counseling Services LLC
New Jersey

Awakening Change Publishing, a subsidiary of

Awakening Change Counseling Services LLC

Post Office Box 8

Voorhees, New Jersey 08043

Reclaiming My Time: A Black Woman's Guide to Self-Care

For information on booking signings, interviews, and other events, please visit www.awakeningchange.org

ISBN: 978-0-578-88642-8

Printed in the United States of America

Table of Contents

Table of Contents

Part I:
Introduction

Reclaim (verb): to retrieve or recover (something previously lost, given, or paid); obtain the return of. (syn: take back, recover, regain)

The definition of 'reclaim' is simple. When you reclaim something like your time, you take it back. It doesn't matter if you lost it, gave it away, or even sold it. Whatever you reclaim, you're taking back ownership.

There's so much power in that word. YOU TAKE IT BACK! No permission required, no explanation needed. If it's yours and you want it back, you take it.

I think that's what Audre Lourde meant when she said "caring for myself is not self-indulgence, it is self-preservation, and that is an act of political warfare". Yes Black woman, the very thought of you caring for your total self - emotionally, physically, intellectually, financially, spiritually, socially, occupationally, and even environmentally - is a violent act of resistance. Because when you find healing, you'll share with your children and they will do the same. When we view self-care as a family heirloom, it becomes the sledgehammer we use to obliterate cycles of multigenerational trauma and destroy generational curses.

You've probably convinced yourself that taking time for yourself is impossible with all you need to accomplish in a day. Your planner is probably full of appointments, deadlines, and reminders for everyone else's stuff except your own.

I get it. We want to be present for the folks in our lives. We take great care in being sure to fully express our love and concern for their safety and well-being. But guess what? If you don't take the time to care for yourself, you won't be around to take care of them.

Maybe you've heard the expression, "you can't pour from an empty cup." Here's the thing: you shouldn't even pour from your cup. Pour from the saucer instead.

Let me explain. When you pour into your own cup, it stays full and eventually begins to overflow, into the saucer beneath it. Your cup is your personal tank. It's filled with all the things that you need to function at optimal levels. If you're constantly pouring out from the cup, you're depleting your resources to provide for others. That's like setting yourself on fire to keep someone else warm.

However, when your cup is always full, to the point of overflow, then you always have something left in the saucer to share with those you love. Pouring from the saucer allows you to be present for others without having to sacrifice yourself in the process.

This is called giving from the overflow, and it isn't selfish. In fact, regular self-care is the most selfless thing you can do.

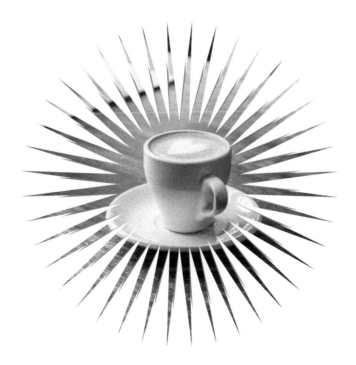

In the chapters that follow, I discuss all of the components of a strong self-care plan and challenge you to put what you're reading into practice. The activities and thought questions throughout this book are intended to help you implement the strategies you'll read about. This book was designed to provide you with an informed action plan.

All you need is an open mind, a pen for taking notes, and the readiness to reclaim your time!

Each chapter features real stories from Black women, just like you. These are women who have faced challenges and overcome them by making their self-care a priority. I also include information to help you understand some of the science that makes "self-care" work.

You've taken an AMAZING step forward just by picking up this book. Whether it was a gift from someone who cares about you, or a decision that you made to make this the year that you live your best life, I'm proud of you for being here. I can't promise you this process will be easy. But I most definitely can guarantee it will be worth it. Every word written here comes from the heart. My goal is to see other Black Women win! We continually face so many challenges, and we typically suffer in silence because we're trying to be strong (we'll talk about that later).

It's our time to speak up and, as Representative Maxine Waters so eloquently stated, reclaim our time. It's time to finally get the healing you deserve.

It's been nearly four years since the (now viral) video of Representative Maxine Waters' iconic phrase, "RECLAIMING MY TIME!" made its rounds on the internet. That powerful phrase immediately made an impact on social media, as Black Women across the world adopted the statement as their new mantra, making a commitment to be unapologetically about their business. It was wonderful to see so many Black women reaffirm their right to exist in the ways that made them the most comfortable.

But, like all viral internet sensations, the conversation seemed to fall dead in the water. Other internet memes soon replaced Auntie Maxine. Numerous tragedies demanded our courage and strength to endure. We had new names to say and remember, new protests to coordinate.

And then there was COVID. *heavy sigh*

When the world came to a screeching halt in March 2020, we were all thrown for a loop. Even if we already had decent self-care and coping skills, many of us began floundering for ways to practice balance and mindfulness and reduce stress amidst the chaos.

Children were sent home for remote learning, and parents found themselves working from home, struggling to juggle multiple roles and manage the new expectations put upon them. This transition was especially hard for some women as they strived to remain present for their children, spouses and partners while managing the growing demands of their primary occupations.

Women have lost the luxury of a daily commute to switch between mom-mode and work-mode and back again. In this new existence, women are simultaneously the teacher's aide, mom, spouse/partner, and employee in the same space and often at the same time.

Even when you finally find a routine that allows some normalcy my bet is that it cost you something.

What did you sacrifice, Sis? Was it a decent night's sleep?   Eating habits? Your exercise routine? Intimacy with your partner? Your meditation practice? What did you lose in the COVID-shuffle? What part of your peace got pushed to the side, or forgotten about altogether, so that you could show up for the important folks in your life?

Take a moment and jot down what these things were. Whatever you gave up, it's time to reclaim it!

As you can see, this isn't your typical self-help book. This book is a combination of information, motivation, worksheets, and journal prompts all designed to start you on the path to consistent self-care. The activities are simple and require very little time or expense because I genuinely believe that self-care shouldn't be another item on your already endless to do list. Self-care should be refreshing and calming, not stressful or overwhelming.

In the chapters that follow, I discuss all of the components of a strong self-care plan and challenge you to put what you're reading into practice. The activities and thought questions throughout this book are intended to help you implement the strategies you'll read about. This book was designed to provide you with an informed action plan.

All you need is an open mind, a pen for taking notes, and the readiness to reclaim your time!

Each chapter features real stories from Black women, just like you. These are women who have faced challenges and overcome them by making their self-care a priority. I also include information to help you understand some of the science that makes "self-care"works.

You've taken an AMAZING step forward just by picking up this book. Whether it was a gift from someone who cares about you, or a decision that you made to make this the year that you live your best life, I'm proud of you for being here. I can't promise you this process will be easy. But I most definitely can guarantee it will be worth it. Every word written here comes from the heart. My goal is to see other Black Women win! We continually face so many challenges, and we typically suffer in silence because we're trying to be strong.

One final note: The information contained in this book is merely a recommendation for how and where to get started. Yes, I am a licensed therapist, but I am not YOUR therapist so I do not know your unique needs. I wrote this book to help you find the motivation to put yourself first - consider it your permission slip for your self-care field trip.

Nothing you read here is a substitute for therapy, and it is strongly recommended that you connect with a licensed therapist to more fully address any emotional distress you may be experiencing. For a listing of Black therapists in your area, check out the resources section (pg. X) or speak with your insurance carrier for a list of in-network providers.

It's our time to speak up and, as Representative Maxine Waters so eloquently stated, reclaim our time. It's time to finally get the healing you deserve. Take a deep breath, grab your favorite pen, and let's begin!

With love,
Tiffany

PERSONAL SACRIFICES

Write down what you gave up during COVID and how it has impacted you mentally, physically and spiritually.

What I gave up	What it cost		
	Mentally	Physically	Spiritually

SETTING INTENTIONS.

Before you continue, take a moment to sit with your thoughts. Think about the reason you picked up this book. What did you hope to gain from reading it? Choose 1-2 sentences that summarize those intentions and write them here.

_____

_____

_____

_____

_____

_____

_____

_____

_____

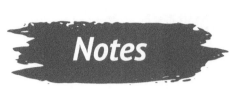

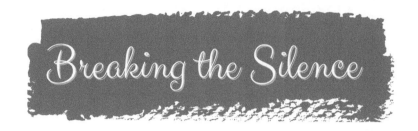

Breaking the Silence

Black Women are less likely to seek professional support (ie therapy) because of the general collective mistrust of the system (that's a whole 'notha book in itself). So what DO Black Women tend to do when they're tired of carrying the burden of strength? We silence ourselves. Yup. We don't take a time out, or put out an SOS. We simply suffer silently.

Oh, but we don't call it that.

We call it being grateful because "it could always be worse" or because "there's someone who has it worse than me" or "I don't want to be a burden."

We find creative ways to bury our frustration, anger, and resentment under the veneer of a smile. In public, we're available and happy, but behind closed doors, we feel like a fraud and we stress about everything falling apart.

We refuse to acknowledge our feelings, choosing instead to focus on the people who "need us."

Any of this sound familiar?

Although these coping mechanisms appear to help us ease the demands of our lives, they actually become unnecessary weights that are keeping us from really soaring as our best selves.

Am I asking you to run away from all your responsibilities and create a new life? No! The fact is even if that were a viable solution, wherever you go, you take YOU with you. A change of scenery won't do much if you don't address the core issues driving you to escape in the first place.

In 'The Color Purple,' Shug Avery sings to Celie "Sistah, you been on my mind oh Sistah we're two of a kind. Sistah, I'm keeping my eye on you."

That's how I feel about you. Yes, you! I'm concerned about the way you make time for everyone in your life, but neglect yourself.

I see you: Tired, frustrated, overwhelmed and still saying yes. You will drop everything at a moment's notice for folks who wouldn't lift a finger for you. You wear the badge and cape of the 'Strong Black Woman' in public while feeling completely powerless in private. You're the strong friend, the one who everyone comes to for advice but rarely does anyone ask how you're feeling - if they ever do at all.

I've been there. It's a lonely and extremely exhausting place to be. The fact is, no matter how desperately you want to get to a better, healthier, happier place, if you don't have a plan it'll never happen.

That was Denise's story. Denise was in her late 20's and, by all outward accounts, BOSS CHICK. She was #GOALS. She had a successful and quite lucrative career, a committed relationship, lots of friends, and a beautiful apartment. It looked like she was living the dream. Whenever anyone called on her - family, friends, coworkers - Denise always said yes. ALWAYS.

She didn't want to disappoint anyone by being unavailable. But Denise was often tired. She was on medication for hypertension, had gained a significant amount of weight in the past 6 months, and felt extremely unfulfilled. Initially, Denise started counseling because she was lacking motivation and worried she may be depressed. It didn't occur to Denise that she was pouring from an empty cup and simply needed to rest and refocus.

Denise started to set and maintain boundaries so that she could reclaim her time. She found the time to schedule appointments for her routine health screenings that were way overdue. She connected with a nutritionist. Denise got back to the gym, and started to see results in her weight loss.

Her sleep improved and her energy increased. She found herself being more creative and, because she wasn't so irritable, anxious, and depressed, she found that her communication had gotten better too. Denise's blood pressure also returned to normal range.

Yes, Denise is a REAL person, not some made up story. And, YES, you can have the same results. But first, you have to take off the cape, Sis. This SuperWoman thing you've got going on looks good on paper, but it's not sustainable. If it was, would you really be reading a book about creating a self-care plan right now?

Are you familiar with the Strong Black Woman trope? Many of us even wear the title like a badge of honor. Historically speaking, it isn't something that we chose. If you go back to the days of slavery, when Black women were raped, their children and spouses sold, and they had no say in the matter, strength wasn't even an option.

We inherited it.

I'm also not saying that being strong is a bad thing. Things get hairy when we refuse to talk about our pain, seek out the help we need, or make the necessary changes out of fear of appearing weak. It's that fear that we need to address, and quickly!

Remember, this is practice. There's no right or wrong way to go about it. You're simply working to create a space that is 100% for you. These suggestions and journal prompts are intended to stimulate deeper thinking around who you are and the things that make you the happiest.

I'm keeping my eye on you. Let's make it work!

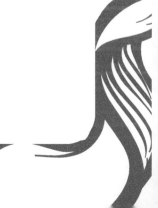

MASKED UP

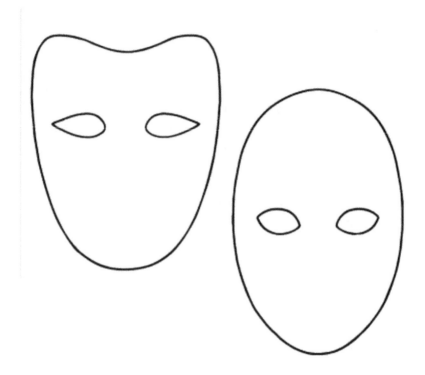

It's time to face your truth. There are 2 masks on this page. The first represents the face that we show to the outside world. Take a moment to reflect. Using words or illustrations, create a visual representation of the face you show the world on the first mask.

The second represents our authentic selves - all of our thoughts, feelings, and frustrations. Again, using words or illustrations, create a visual representation of the face you keep hidden.

Then, take a moment to reflect on both masks.

How do the outside and inside aspects of you relate to each other?

_____

_____

_____

_____

_____

Did you learn or rediscover anything about yourself? If yes, what?

_____

_____

_____

_____

_____

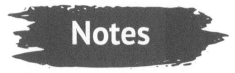

Notes

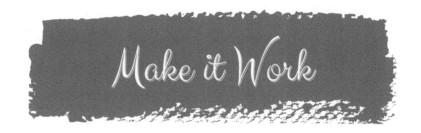

Make it Work

Typically, when I introduce self-care to my clients the first excuse I hear is, "I don't have enough time for all that!" But, if you sit down and take an honest look at what you do on an average day, you'd be surprised to find you've got more time than you think. Don't believe me? OK, bet! Let me explain.

Think of every hour as a dollar. You start each week with $168 in your bank account. The account can't go into overdraft and balances can't be carried over. Your withdrawals are based on what you do each day.

For example, if you get six hours of sleep every night for seven days $42 would be deducted from your account. If you work eight hours a day for five days a week, that would take $40 from your account And so on, for every activity of every day of your week (getting the kids to practice, fixing dinner, packing lunches, etc.).

Tally your 'expenses' for the week, and subtract them from your starting budget to see what's left over.

Self-Care Calculator

Starting Balance	168.0
ACTIVITY	# OF HOURS PER WEEK
SLEEP	56
MEALS/MEAL PREP	10
COMMUTE	4
WORK	50
GYM	0
SCHOOL/COURSEWORK	15
SPIRITUALITY	1
LAUNDRY	3
GROCERY SHOPPING	3
SOCIAL TIME	10
TOTAL	152
AVAILABLE TIME (Starting balance - Total) =	16

At first, that number may look large to you. You might think, "there's no way that I have THAT much time left over every week."

I assure you, you probably do. You're probably filling that time with mindless distractions that could be repurposed for your self-care routine. Think about it.

How much time do you spend scrolling through social media?

Playing video games?

Scrolling on the internet with no real purpose?

All of that time is time that you can reclaim.

The issue isn't that the time isn't there. The real issue is what you need to make the most of what you have. You need to stop making excuses and start making real changes.
Excuses are easy to find:
"I'm tired."
"I don't feel like it"

But if you keep doing what you've always done, you're going to keep getting the same results.

Aren't you tired of having low energy, being unhappy and unfulfilled? You opened this book because you wanted to stop the cycle of being overworked, overwhelmed, and underappreciated.
Right now, you're the poster child for the Strong Black Woman stereotype. But, Sis, I don't want you faking the funk to appear strong.

I want you to really BE strong.

You have a choice. You can have this stressed out, overwhelmed, and ultimately fake life. Or you can start living your absolute best life.

It won't be easy. Both choices will be difficult; you either keep going on the way you have, or you begin making even small changes. I'll give you that.

But you have to decide which hard choice you're willing to live with. The hard that you're in right now (burning the candle at both ends, not taking care of yourself, not living your best life) is not sustainable. If you don't make serious changes soon, your health will be negatively affected (if it's not already) and your loved ones will be burying you!

The "hard" that I'm challenging you to step into actually gets easier with practice. With every step you take towards creating the space for yourself, you actually extend your life. You'll be adding more time to fulfill your purpose, to find happiness, and to improve the overall quality of your life. Sis, you have to make it work.

You might be saying, "how do I put this stuff into practice? I don't know where to start." **The truth is, if you're still reading, you've already gotten started**. You made an intentional decision to be still and do something for yourself.

In the chapters that follow, we're going to define wellness and self-care and identify ways you can be intentional with your schedule. We'll also build your communication skills and exercise setting boundaries so that you can maintain the plan you establish for yourself.

We'll start small and before you know it, you will have created a lifestyle where you have so much more to give the folks that you care about because you've learned to put yourself first.

You see, self-care isn't selfish.

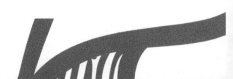

Here's the "tea". *The best way to care for the people you love is to care for yourself first! If you're not okay. They're not going to be okay:*

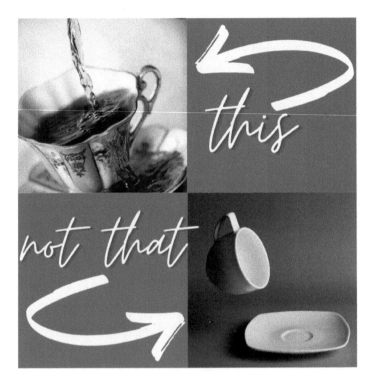

Not enough money

Another excuse people use regarding self-care is lack of money."Well, I would love to take care of myself, but you know I got bills to pay."

"I would love to treat myself, but the kids need x, y, and z."

This one is easily put to bed. You don't need extra cash to take care of yourself. The strategies we will focus on use what you already have to make positive changes in every area of your life.

Do not go out and start spending money that you don't have for some project that you know you're not going to finish and create stress that you don't have the capacity to deal with. (Read that again!)

Start small, start where you are, with what you have, and watch the difference that a little bit makes. Self-care shouldn't hurt. It shouldn't cause stress, and it shouldn't cause a major disruption to your life. Self-care adds value to your life. It helps you care for, uplift, celebrate, encourage, and support yourself in becoming the best version of your authentic self.

You don't need a lot of money or a lot of time to implement a good self-care plan - you just need to be intentional. Small goals make big progress. In the chapters ahead I'm going to teach you how to set achievable goals that will increase your likelihood of success. We'll establish accountability and create a safe space where you can thrive.

The point isn't to be perfect. It's about being authentic and making good progress. The first thing you'll need to do is make the time for a meaningful self care practice. Trust me, the time is there. You just have to set it aside.

After you set your schedule, you'll learn the 8 dimensions of wellness and how they relate to your plan. That's where the magic happens. You'll use what you've learned to begin an intentional journey of self-exploration designed to deepen your self-care practice.

SELF-CARE CALCULATOR

Use this chart to calculate how much time you have available for self-care activities in an average week. Be completely honest with your answers. You can't fix what you don't face. Besides, no one is going to see this, and if you can't be honest with yourself, what's the point?

There are no right or wrong answers. This activity is designed to help you to learn more about yourself and find the time to practice self-care.

At the top of the chart, you'll see a 'starting balance' of 168. That represents the number of hours in a week. We all have the same number of hours in the day.

Along the left-hand side, you'll see some activities that typically consume your daily schedule. In each of the corresponding columns, calculate how many hours per week you spend doing each activity.

Add up all your totals and then subtract the grand total from your starting balance. That number is how much time you spend on your obligations.

Self-Care Calculator

Starting Balance	168.0
ACTIVITY	# OF HOURS PER WEEK
SLEEP	
MEALS/MEAL PREP	
COMMUTE	
WORK	
GYM	
SCHOOL/COURSEWORK	
SPIRITUALITY	
LAUNDRY	
GROCERY SHOPPING	
SOCIAL TIME	
TOTAL	
AVAILABLE TIME (Starting balance - Total) =	

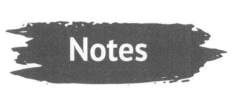

Notes

Part II:

Living Well or Walking Dead?

I want you to think about the last zombie movie you watched. Was it an old school zombie movie where the zombies moved at a slow crawl, or was it something like World War Z super-powered zombies zooming around very quickly. What's the same in every zombie movie is that no matter how life-like the zombies move or sound, they're actually shells of who they used to be. They're not really alive, even though their physical bodies continue to move forward.

When we don't keep a consistent and dedicated practice of self-care, we become like zombies. We're not ourselves anymore. We're not really alive, but we're not completely dead. We're walking dead.

That's pretty scary! It's not something any of us would aspire to.

Now, contrast that with the survivors in zombie movies. The survivors are usually doing what they can to take care of themselves - to stay safe. Whether it's finding food, shelter, or supplies, they're dedicated to self-preservation.

Compare your self-care, right now, right at this moment, to the characters in a zombie movie. Are you a zombie – not quite dead, but definitely not alive? A ghoul that everyone runs from in terror? Or are you a survivor - fully functioning and able to take care of yourself even when there's chaos around you?

Yes, even in the chaos you can practice self-care. That's where we've got it twisted. We think that if we're practicing self-care, we'll never stress again and that's simply not true. We'll still face stress, but we'll know how to deal with it. Just like survivors in zombie movies.

What does the zombie version of you look like?

_____

_____

_____

_____

_____

What does the survivor version of you look like?

_____

_____

_____

_____

_____

What tools or resources does the survivor version of you possess that the zombie version does not?

_____

_____

_____

_____

Eight Dimensions of Wellness

Living well happens when we make consistent practice of caring for ourselves that encompasses all of the eight dimensions of wellness. Yes, I know it sounds like a lot, but before you say "I don't have time" refer back to the self-care calculator from Chapter Three. You have the time, Sis!

Adjust your thinking, be intentional, and put yourself on a schedule. The eight dimensions of wellness are much easier than you think especially because of the overlap between dimensions.

In Part II, we'll walk through each dimension and use activities to help you create a plan for yourself in each area.

DO NOT RUSH THIS PROCESS.

Take time to work intentionally through each section. Be brutally honest with yourself. Give yourself permission to be vulnerable and ask for help when you need it. While this is a 'self-help' book, many of these activities are most effective when reviewed with a therapist for greater insight and accountability.

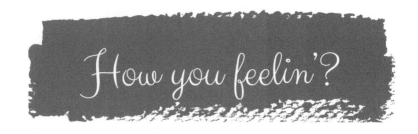
How you feelin'?

~Emotional Wellness~

Emotional wellness, simply put, is being aware of your feelings and having positive ways to express them. But what exactly are emotions and feelings?

One explanation is that your **emotions are thoughts that you can feel**. After all, feelings are triggered by a thought, or experience. You didn't "just snap!" You may not know the reason in the moment, but there's definitely a trigger, or multiple triggers depending on the situation.

The following example shows how triggers affect our emotions. Let's say you leave home later than expected, hit traffic, and log in for work later than expected. Shortly after you begin work, your boss calls and asks you to clear your afternoon calendar for a meeting.

You immediately think that you're going to be reprimanded or, even worse, terminated. You have a good record, you know isn't your usual behavior, but you begin to panic as soon as the call's over. Your panic makes you snap at coworkers as a headache creeps up the back of your neck. Now you're anxious, struggling to concentrate, and your patience is paper thin.

Sis, you're an emotional wreck! Let's figure out how to get you together.

We'll start with the triggering event: your boss asking you to clear your schedule. While you may have been annoyed by the morning commute, ultimately it was the phone call that set your anxiety in motion. We'll talk about that morning rush a little bit later.

That call triggers the negative thought that you're going to be reprimanded or fired, your body physically aligns with that idea. The tension in your neck and anxiety you feel are in direct relationship with the notion of being in trouble. Your fear response causes you to react in a closed off and cold way (you may even be triggering your coworkers). When you're not aware of the cycle, you become a bull in a China shop, destroying everything in your path.

But what if the meeting was a request for you to join a special project? How much energy and time was wasted being anxious? You allowed a negative experience from outside of work – a schedule issue and traffic jam – to put you in a heightened state of arousal so that left you easily triggered until you "just snapped" at anyone who spoke to you.

In life, it's not always as simple as a traffic jam or unexpected meeting. You may have a history of trauma that shapes the way that you interact with the world around you. Perhaps you've experienced discrimination in your workplace and are now extremely uncomfortable in certain environments. It doesn't matter what the noise and triggers are – what matters is what you do about them.

Practicing emotional self-care will require you to identify your triggers and automatic thoughts, and then choose healthier responses. Books like this one can be useful in beginning the process, but professional help is strongly advised. We can't always see through our own stuff so having an unbiased accountability partner to assist us is one of the most "self-care" things we can do for ourselves.

One small way to start addressing your triggers is with a journal. Commit to writing down your thoughts and feelings when you're feeling angry or upset, then waiting a day before you respond.

OH SNAP!

Think about the last time you "just snapped."
What triggered you? Go over the situation and
complete the chart with as much detail as you can
remember.

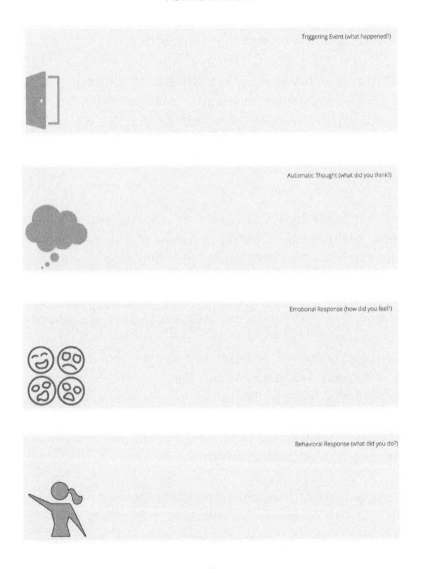

Triggering Event (what happened?)

Automatic Thought (what did you think?)

Emotional Response (how did you feel?)

Behavioral Response (what did you do?)

Rate your reaction to the situation on a scale of 1-10; with 1 being a poor emotional reaction, and 10 the best possible reaction. _____

Explain why you gave yourself that score.

_____

_____

_____

_____

_____

_____

What's ONE thing you can do to improve your score?

_____

_____

_____

_____

_____

Consider sharing your responses with a therapist who can assist you with implementing a plan to improve in this area.

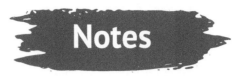

Notes

Prayer Only Works If You Do

~Spiritual Wellness~

Spiritual wellness speaks to the ways in which we connect to others, through a sense of community, and to our higher purpose. Although religion can be how we express our spirituality, there is a difference.

In the simplest terms Spirituality represents connection, while Religion is the set of defined practices that can guide connections with others.

Research shows that spirituality helps reduce feelings of depression, improve self-esteem, and increase overall life satisfaction. And, if you're a practicing member of a faith, the time you spend in "fellowship" can boost your mood and give you additional support to navigate life's difficulties.

There are multiple benefits to having a self-care routine with a strong spiritual component, but there are also dangers in over-spiritualizing your self-care.

If you're a person of faith, it's easy to trust that your Higher Power will just 'handle it' a la Olivia Pope. Unfortunately, life rarely works that way. You still have your part to do. You have to be intentional with meditation and prayer, when applying spiritual principles in your day-to-day life.

Even if you don't ascribe to organized religion, but instead rely on guidance from ancestors, you still have a job to do. You have to be still and listen. You have to diligently watch for lessons from the Universe. Nothing just happens on its own.

Your Higher Power is the source of your energy, creativity, power, confidence, EVERYTHING. It's the electrical socket. You are the plug. **You must make the effort to connect to your source on a regular basis in order to have what you need.**

CREATING CONNECTION

Identify one activity that fills your spiritual cup. It can be anything - meditation, prayer, yoga, dance, a card reading - so long as it connects you with your Higher Power/Higher Purpose. Find a quiet space and engage in that activity for at least 15 minutes. Record any messages you may have received.

_____

_____

_____

_____

_____

_____

_____

_____

_____

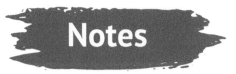

Notes

Beauty & Brains

~Intellectual Wellness~

We rarely consider learning as synonymous with wellness, but enriching the mind has many benefits. The intellectual dimension of our self-care plan is concerned with expanding your knowledge, skills, and creative expression. The goal of intellectual wellness is to help us to grow through our experiences by keeping our minds sharp. There are countless ways to achieve this, but we'll focus on reading, learning a new skill or language, and travel.

The most easily accessible tool for nurturing our intellect is a good book. Whether you prefer an audio book, tablet, or hard copy, the main benefit of books is that they actively engage our brains. We have to pay attention and keep up to maintain the experience. Whatever your favorite genre, a book expands your mind to people, places, and things outside of your norm. Bonus points if you can have stimulating conversation about what you're reading and hear other opinions and perspectives. (Book club, anyone?).

The current digital age makes learning a new language or skill a click away. Masterclasses that can teach you anything from growing your own vegetables to writing your first novel are available on a variety of platforms. And let's not forget YouTube University where you can learn practically anything. Decide what you want to learn, and the knowledge is literally at your fingertips.

Travel is another way to stretch your intellectual limits while having a ton of fun. Travel is more than sitting on the beach in reflective contemplation (although that's cool for your emotional, spiritual, and environmental self care).

When you travel, aim to be intentional in absorbing the cultures and traditions of the people in that location. Have a discussion about some of the differences between your locations and attempt to learn the language.

The goal of intellectual well-being is to prompt your own growth. You are taking steps to break free from unhealthy patterns and learn new ones. Congrats!

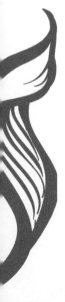

LEVEL UP YOUR LEARNING

1. Identify a topic you'd like to learn more about over the next 30 days. Spend 15 minutes writing down all of your questions about that topic.

2. Review your questions. Rank them by your level in each. For example, if you have 10 questions, number one will be the question you are MOST interested in and number ten will be the question you are least interested in finding the answer to right now. It doesn't need to be spot on, you just need to get organized enough to start the process.

3. Highlight your top three. Order them by which answer would lead to the next.

4. Where are you likely to find the information that will help you to answer those questions?

5. Grab your calendar/planner.

6. Schedule ten days of research for each of the three questions you selected.

In thirty days, you will have expanded your knowledge in a particular area.

Congratulations!

Topic:

What do I want to know?

Where can I find the answers I'm looking for (resources)?:

What have I learned?:

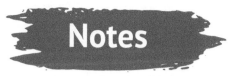

Notes

Sleeping Beauty

~Physical Wellness~

When most people think of taking care of themselves, they instantly think of their physical needs – healthy diet, regular exercise, and personal grooming.

Most of the time, when I ask clients about a self-care plan, their responses fall into this dimension (and usually nowhere else). Ladies, while we enjoy our manicure, pedicures and spa days, a commitment to self-care is more than that.

According to Center for Disease Control (CDC) statistics, 44% of African American women over the age of 20 have hypertension and had a life expectancy that was shorter than their White counterparts. In fact, the only group with a shorter life expectancy was Black men (2018 Health, United Stated Data Finder). Additional statistics suggest that Black women are more likely to die from heart disease or cancer than old age or accidental death. The data shows not only are we living shorter lives, but quality of living (on average) is not so great. We must reclaim our health if we want to be around to see the next generation.

You don't need to run out and get a gym membership and a trainer or, swear off carbs. Not only is that drastic, but it's also not sustainable. Start with small changes, Sis. If your job requires you to sit for most of your day, try standing up to stretch for one minute every hour. If you're always on your feet, it can be helpful to have the proper footwear and take regular breaks. Take breath breaks throughout the day to get your oxygen flowing.

A quick five minute meditation (which also counts as your spiritual and emotional self-care) can help your body function more efficiently.

One of the most overlooked components of physical wellness, though, is sleep. The adage, "you can rest when you're dead" isn't exactly the mantra you should live by – ESPECIALLY as a Black woman. The National Heart, Lung, and Blood Institute defines sleep deficiency as a condition that occurs "if you have one or more of the following: you don't get enough sleep, you sleep at the wrong time (out of sync with your body's natural rhythm), you don't sleep well or you have a sleep disorder."

If you're over the age of 18, you need 7-8 hours of sleep per night to function at optimal levels. What are optimal levels? Well, let's look at all the things your body does while you sleep: repairs your heart and blood vessels (great for healing the effects of blood pressure), restores brain function (this improves your mood and thinking), and even regulates hormones that cause you to feel hungry (helps in weight loss efforts). Compare the list of sleep benefits with the list of disease risks and I think you'll see where I'm going with this.

Contrary to what you've been told (i.e "you can sleep when you're dead") you absolutely do need to rest. I know you think you need to work overtime for extra cash to cover expenses, but that's just not true. In fact, by trying to maintain an insane schedule, you're burning yourself out, and eventually you will crash. You cannot rob your body of the fuel it needs and think that one massage and a glass of wine will help it bounce back. That's not how this works.

All the spa days in the world are no substitute for a great night's sleep. Commit to developing a soothing nighttime routine that helps you to wind down and get a replenishing night's sleep. Everything else in your self-care plan will depend on it.

Environmental factors can play a huge role in helping you to get a proper night's rest. First, make sure your bedroom is a comfortable temperature. If you typically run hot, lower the thermostat at bedtime or keep a fan on your nightstand. Next, eliminate as much artificial light as possible. Your brain interprets the light from your electronic devices as daylight and will think that it's time to be awake and alert. Try to turn everything off at least 30 minutes before bedtime.

Consider charging your phone away from your bedside to reduce the urge for late night scrolling through social media. If you have a diffuser, essential oils like lavender and chamomile can be excellent aids for drifting into a peaceful rest. What you do isn't as important as being consistent - so identify the routine that works for you and enjoy your beauty sleep.

GO TO SLEEP!

Good sleep is the BEST gift you can give yourself. But it rarely just happens - you have to create an environment that primes your body for maximum rest. Think about your nighttime routine. Do you just fall into bed exhausted from the day or are you intentionally winding down each evening? For the next seven nights, try to be intentional about quieting your mind and relaxing your body as you prepare for sleep.

Here's one way to start.

1. Lay down in a comfortable position and take three deep cleansing breaths.
2. Starting from your feet, tense and relax all of the muscles of your body one group at a time (feet and ankles, knees and calves, thighs and pelvic muscles, abdomen and lower back, arms and hands, shoulders and neck, even your face).
3. Take three more deep cleansing breaths.

Sweet dreams!

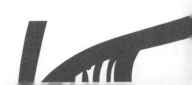

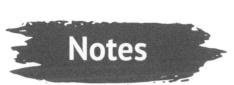

Notes

My Space

~Environmental Wellness~

Environmental wellness focuses on your surroundings. The goal is to create spaces that stimulate health and well-being, which also promote connection and interaction with others. Your environmental self-care plan should include intentional boundaries to protect your peace. In this case, the boundaries are more physical than emotional or social (we'll discuss those important boundaries later).

Do you have a clutter-free space for yourself, that's peaceful, and inviting? If so, when was the last time you were there? How does the space make you feel? What items in the space add to your feelings?

Don't have such a space? Create it! Even if it's only a corner in your bedroom, claiming a small space can make a huge difference. Be intentional about what you put there. Set clear boundaries around what and who will be allowed in your space and notice any changes in your mood and mindset.

Another piece for your environmental wellness toolbox is time spent in nature. You don't need to start camping or hiking every weekend. You simply need to go outside. Sunlight is the greatest source of Vitamin D available to us, and SIS! Vitamin D is BAE!

Research shows that Vitamin D boosts your immune system and is helpful for treating and even PREVENTING some forms of cancer, osteoporosis, rheumatoid arthritis, multiple sclerosis, hypertension, heart disease, obesity, and a host of mood disorders.

The very things that lower Black women's life expectancy are treated with Vitamin D. That alone makes sunshine worth adding to our self-care routine.

It's worth noting that environmental self-care is tied to physical, spiritual, emotional, and even social self-care as well. Self-care doesn't need to be complex. You can feed your emotional, physical, and environmental needs just by taking a walk.

Get creative and see how many activities you can identify that check multiple boxes. Remember, we're trying to reclaim our time, not fill our schedules with never-ending to-dos.

FINDING MY HAPPY PLACE

For each season, identify two (2) activities that you can do outdoors. Try to think of at least one freebie so you're not limited by finances.

Winter

- _____

- _____

Spring

- _____

- _____

Summer

- _____

- _____

Fall

- _____

- _____

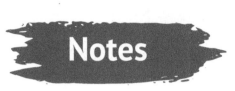

Notes

Money Moves

~Financial Wellness~

Just the mention of finances can be a major stressor, I know. But, the thing is, if you don't face it, you won't fix it. And honestly, money is one thing everyone could use a little more of. So, let's put on our big girl pants and have a hard conversation about getting financial wellness.

In her book, "You Are A Badass at Making Money," Jenn Sincero writes, "your thoughts inspire emotions that inspire action that forms your 'reality.'"

She says, and I agree, that until you're clear on your thoughts about money, you'll never be able to break away from your dysfunctional relationship with it. Your experiences with money shape your thoughts and feelings about finances.

If your family was financially stable, you may have grown up with strong examples of money management financial responsibility. By contrast, if you were raised in a home where money was scarce, you may not even have heard finances being discussed, but you knew there wasn't enough. Either experience would significantly shape someone's perspective on finances and how they interact with money.

The first step to financial wellness is to figure out what you think about money. Reflect on conversations about money that took place in your home when you were growing up. (how many times did you hear, "We ain't got McDonald's money!"

I know I can't begin to count!) You probably have some strong emotional reactions to discussions about money that are directly impacting your financial reality. Unpacking those emotions will unlock the keys to developing your financial self-care plan.

Every plan will be different. If you realize that you've been spending too much a budget may be useful. Your plan could be to find the budget that fits your lifestyle. Maybe your issue is that you haven't been saving for retirement, or secured life insurance because you have anxiety about the future.

Addressing that anxiety will be essential to your financial wellness plan. It's tempting to use a budget calculator to cut your spending and increase your savings, but if financial wellness was that simple, wouldn't everyone be doing it? True financial wellness can only be achieved when you address the influencing issues.

MONEY MINDSET

Think back to conversations around money in your home as you were growing up. How many of those conversations were positive? How many were negative? Which ideas about money have you retained? The answers to these questions will help you identify what's holding you back.

Next, we'll challenge your negative beliefs about money. Review your previous answers and rewrite them as affirmations to create a more positive perspective on your finances. Repeat your affirmations daily to shift your money mindset.

Use these examples to get you started:

> **What I was taught:** Money doesn't buy happiness.
>
> **The remix:** Money doesn't buy happiness, BUT money does allow me to fund the activities that make me happy. Without money, I cannot provide basic necessities for my family (food, clothing, shelter, etc) or do things that are fun.
>
> **Affirmation:** Money creates opportunities for me to do the things that make me happy.

> **What I was taught:** The love of money is the root of all evil.
>
> **The remix:** A desire to be financially stable does not equate to a love of money. I can have a desire to be financially stable without compromising my morals, ethics, and/or values.
>
> **Affirmation:** I love myself and my family enough to ensure that we have what we need. Financial stability helps me to meet those needs.

What I was taught:

_____

_____

_____

The remix:

_____

_____

_____

Affirmation:

_____

_____

_____

What I was taught:

_____

_____

_____

The remix:

_____

_____

_____

Affirmation:

_____

_____

_____

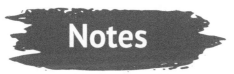

Notes

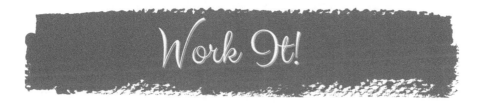

~Occupational Wellness~

In an average week, many of us spend more time at work than anywhere else. If you work from home, the lines between work time and downtime can get significantly blurred. For this reason occupational wellness is a vital part of a complete self-care plan. This isn't only about your job. It's about gaining personal satisfaction from both your work and your hobbies - essentially, the work-life balance that so many of us seek.

The truth is, it's less of a balance and more like a rhythm. Some days, you'll have project deadlines or special events that require more time and attention, and that's ok. Your focus here should be finding your groove. Try to be as intentional about engaging with your hobbies and interests as you are about meeting work related deadlines.

As we explore occupational wellness, let's begin with job satisfaction. Think about where you are in your career and ask yourself the following: Do you feel stuck in your current role? Are you ready to move on, but not sure how? Are you considering entrepreneurship, but afraid to take the plunge?

Whatever the change you need - set a goal, create a plan, and do it! Most of your waking hours are spent at work. Why not do something that you love? Life is too short to be miserable - especially about something you have the power to change.

Occupational wellness overlaps with intellectual wellness because improving your career begins with improving your knowledge. What must you know before you make the career leap of your daydreams? What connections need to be made? How can you reposition yourself to be ready for the opportunity when it presents itself? These are questions you need to reflect on as you reach for occupational wellness.

Now, about those hobbies. You might not even remember what it's like to actually have hobbies – and no, a side hustle doesn't count. Hobbies are activities that help us to decompress from our obligations and refill our cups. We do hobbies purely for pleasure and at our leisure. Hobbies don't demand deadlines. There are no invoices. It's you and your peace.

Your hobby may be gardening, coloring, enjoying a good cup of something awesome (tea, coffee, wine, whatever!) with a good friend, or even some time spent in quiet solitude. When's the last time you did something simply for your own satisfaction? If you have to think about it, it's been WAY TOO LONG!

Remember, the goal with occupational wellness isn't balance - that would imply that everything is equal at all times. Your goal is rhythm, to find your groove. Some days might be a classic R&B slow dance, while others will feel more like Jersey House music. You just have to feel the beat and move your feet.

FIND YOUR RHYTHM

1. Make a list of all of the hobbies that you have (or would like to have).

_____

_____

_____

_____

2. Highlight activities you have all the tools for and could begin right now.

3. Now, grab your planner. Look at your work schedule and any upcoming deadlines you may have. Based on this week's schedule, where can you set aside thirty minutes for your hobbies? Make an appointment with yourself to do that activity at least once this week.

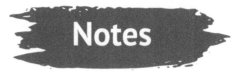

Notes

Drawing the Line

~Social Wellness~

When we are socially well, we feel connected and supported. We have a sense of belonging and feel safe. Sounds simple enough. But social wellness can be challenging because it requires us to create boundaries. Enforcing those boundaries with folks who aren't so good for us can be complicated.

You may already be thinking of a few people whose company is more like work than relaxation. Sometime, when you're seen as the "strong friend" or the family member who "has it all together" spending time with others can be draining. Of course you love your friends and family, but you also need time to yourself, and they rarely understand that. Even worse, when you try to fall back, you're accused of "acting funny" or thinking "you're better than everybody else." Sound familiar?

We teach people how to treat us so the reality is that you've trained these people to depend on you so much. BUT! Just like you taught them before, you can teach them something different. As Kevin Hart said, "You gon' learn today!" Part of the whole Strong Black woman persona is always being available for everyone else and putting your needs and feelings on the back burner. In order to walk in FULL STRENGTH and find social wellness, you're going to have to accept two truths.

Truth #1: "Boundaries" is not a dirty word.
Truth #2: No is a complete sentence.

Let's start with boundaries. Although many people feel like setting boundaries is being mean, the truth is our boundaries protect us and others.

Think about your home. It doesn't matter if you live in a single-family house or an apartment, you pay for a certain amount of space. You're responsible only for what happens in that space. If your neighbors throw a wild party and completely trash their living room, you don't lose your security deposit or have to pay for repairs. Similarly, if your toilet overflows and ruins the flooring, you wouldn't expect your neighbors to come in and fix it. Why? Because it's not their stuff.

Emotional boundaries work the same way - they are property lines that help us to determine what is our responsibility and what belongs to someone else.

Secondly, no is a complete sentence.

Saying no is the part of self-care we don't talk about enough. If you're working on making the time to care for yourself, you need to learn to say no. You don't have to be a jerk about it. Just say no.

For folks who are not used to you refusing their requests, being told no is likely to cause some pretty severe reactions. That's no reason to back off of your boundary. On the contrary, it's more reason to be firm. Remember what I said about teaching people how to treat you? If you keep changing up, no one is going to take you seriously. They'll learn that this is your new dance: ask, get rejected, throw a tantrum, get a yes. Is that the lesson you're trying to teach? **The fact is, givers need to clearly and consistently set boundaries because the takers never will.**

BLURRED LINES

As you were reading, could you identify situations where you need to more clearly assert boundaries? What were those areas? Be as specific as you can.

_____

_____

_____

_____

_____

What would you like your boundaries to look like with those people or situations you identified above.

_____

_____

_____

_____

_____

Consider sharing your responses with your therapist. Your difficulty with establishing clear boundaries may be a sign of other issues that you could use some additional support to work through.

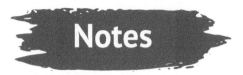

Notes

Part III:

Use A Lifeline

You made it! You've just learned how important it is to take care of yourself, and done some deep digging to identify the areas of your life that your self care plan needs to address.

So, now what? I don't want you to put this book away and go back to busy-ness (no, that's not a typo) as usual. The hardest part of forming a new habit is always getting started, and you've proven to yourself that you can do that. You've jump started an amazing journey of self-exploration and self-love that doesn't need to end when the last page is turned. You owe it to yourself to keep this process going.

If you've ever watched the game show, "Who Wants to be a Millionaire" you know about lifelines. Whenever a contestant is stumped by a question or just wants to be sure, they have the option to use one of four lifelines - ask the audience, phone a friend, 50:50, or ask the host. Rarely, if ever has a contestant made it to the million without using any of their lifelines.

The same is true about your self-care journey - we all need help to reach our goals. This book, though a lifeline of sorts, is only the beginning. Although you've started to dig deep and have hopefully had some AHA! moments, the truth is we're not always completely honest with ourselves. Sometimes, we need an outside perspective to help us reach our goals. Sometimes we need to phone a friend.

In this case, the friend I'm referring to is a therapist. Before you start with the whole "I'm not telling a stranger all my business" excuse hear me out.

First, that "stranger" is legally bound to keep all of the information you share with him or her completely private. That means if they spill the tea, you're rolling in the dough. You don't have that guarantee with your current circle of friends or family regardless of how tight you think you are. Secondly, if you're struggling with asking for help from friends and family because you think you're burdening them with your problems, a therapist is your best option. You can get the support you need without feeling guilty about adding to someone else's sorrows and you don't have to worry about them judging you or throwing what you've shared back in your face. And, most importantly, you don't have to be "crazy" to see a therapist. Going to therapy doesn't mean you're broken or you don't have faith in your Higher Power. It simply means you're committed to becoming the best possible version of yourself. It means you don't just want to LOOK strong on the outside, you want to BE strong!

Therapy is the ultimate way to reclaim your time AND there are a number of resources that can connect you to a Black therapist (check out the resources chapter).

If you've never connected with a therapist before, you may not be sure which questions to ask or how to find the right 'fit.' Here are my suggestions on finding the therapist that's right for you..

1. **Visit their website.** When you read through their information does anything connect with you? Does it feel like they're speaking directly to you and how you think and feel? If yes, this is a great first sign. Consider scheduling a consultation appointment.

2. **Try before you buy!** One of the biggest mistakes you can make is thinking that you HAVE TO stick with the first person who calls you back. NOPE! You have to feel comfortable if you're going to do the work so take your time and choose the therapist that works for you.

3. **Ask questions!** Your consultation is an opportunity for you to interview the therapist to determine if they're the right fit. Ask about more than availability and insurance. What do you need to know in order to feel comfortable?

4.   **Check your benefits.** Review your coverage with your insurance company. In many cases, there is a website on the back of your insurance card that will allow you to access a provider directory. In addition to your medical insurance, you may be eligible for the Employee Assistance Program (EAP) at your job. Using these benefits can significantly lower your out of pocket costs for therapy expenses.

5.   **Be honest!** This may seem obvious, but it's worth reiterating. The more honest you can be about what you're thinking and feeling, the more likely you are to actually benefit from your time in therapy. Resist the urge to look like you have it all together. Remember, the goal is to BE STRONG not just act like it.

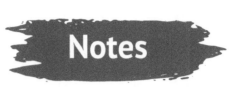

Notes

Resources

Looking for a therapist?
Check out these directories

- **Therapy for Black Girls**
    www.therapyforblackgirls.com

    ○

- **Clinicians of Color Directory**
    www.cliniciansofcolor.org

    ○

- **TheraTribe**
    www.theratribe.com

    ○

- **Black Female Therapists**
    www.blackfemaletherapists.com

    ○

- **Melanin & Mental Health**
    www.melaninandmentalhealth.com

    ○

Epilogue

I hope this workbook has inspired you to take
better care of yourself and maybe even connect
with a therapist.
I'd love to hear your feedback!
Feel free to reach out at
www.awakeningchange.org
and join the mailing list to receive special offers
and discounts.

If you've found this book useful, please leave a
review on goodreads.com or Amazon.com so we
can spread the word that self-care isn't selfish and
help our sisters to reclaim their time as well.

About the Author

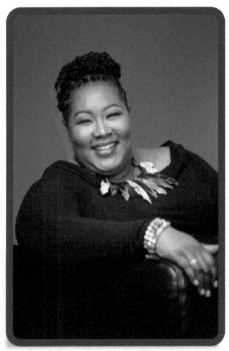

Dr. Tiffany M. Jenkins ("Dr. J") is the founder of Awakening Change Counseling Services LLC located in Cherry Hill, New Jersey. She is licensed as a professional mental health counselor and as a licensed substance abuse counselor and has served in the behavioral health field for over 20 years. As a licensed therapist, Dr. Jenkins works to help "strong friends" find the comfort and support they need and deserve. Dr. Jenkins has been praised for her down-to-earth approach to therapy that assists her clients with making meaningful change in an atmosphere that feels like speaking with an old friend. Dr. Jenkins is proud of her clinical accomplishments, but is most proud of her roles as wife and mom.